Homeopathy Health Guide for Beginners

Knowing The Importance of Homeopathy

By

Henry Duncraig

Copyright@2023

Table of Contents

CHAPTER 1
Introduction

1.1 What is Homeopathy?

Homeopathy is a holistic system of alternative medicine that dates back over two centuries and is based on the fundamental principle of "like cures like." This means that a substance that can cause symptoms in a healthy person can be used in a highly diluted form to treat similar symptoms in a sick individual. The term "homeopathy" itself is derived from the Greek words "homoios" (meaning similar) and "pathos" (meaning suffering or disease), reflecting this core concept.

At the heart of homeopathy is the idea that the body has an innate ability to heal itself. Homeopathic remedies are prepared by serially diluting natural substances, such as plants, minerals, and animal products, and then vigorously shaking the solution at each dilution step, a process known as potentization. This process is believed to release the vital energy or "vital force" of the substance while removing its toxic properties. Homeopathic remedies are usually administered in the form of small, sweet-tasting pellets or liquid solutions.

One of the key principles of homeopathy is individualization. Homeopaths believe that each person is unique, and the same illness can manifest differently in different individuals. Therefore, treatment is tailored to the specific symptoms, emotional state, and overall constitution of the patient. This holistic approach takes into account not only the physical symptoms but also the mental and emotional aspects of a person's health.

Homeopathy is a safe and gentle form of medicine, making it suitable for people of all ages, including infants and pregnant women. It is often used as a complementary therapy alongside conventional medicine, but some individuals also choose to use it as a standalone treatment.

1.2 History of Homeopathy

The history of homeopathy can be traced back to the late 18th century when it was developed by Samuel Hahnemann, a German physician, and chemist. Hahnemann was dissatisfied with the harsh and often ineffective medical practices of his time, such as bloodletting and the use of toxic substances like mercury. This dissatisfaction led him to explore alternative methods of healing.

Hahnemann's breakthrough came when he conducted a series of experiments on himself, taking small doses of quinine, a substance known for causing symptoms similar to those of malaria. To his surprise, he developed symptoms resembling malaria. This observation led him to formulate the principle of "like cures like," which became the foundation of homeopathy.

Over the years, Hahnemann refined his ideas and developed a system of medicine based on his principles. He also introduced the concept of potentization, which involves diluting and succussing (shaking) remedies to increase their healing power while minimizing their toxicity.

Homeopathy gained popularity in Europe during the 19th century and soon spread to other parts of the world. It was particularly embraced in the United States, where it became an established form of healthcare and was widely used by physicians and the general public alike.

Despite facing criticism and skepticism from some quarters of the medical establishment, homeopathy has endured and continues to be practiced today by millions of people worldwide. Its long history is a testament to its perceived efficacy and its ability to resonate with those seeking gentle, individualized, and holistic approaches to health and healing.

1.3 How Homeopathy Works

Homeopathy operates on several fundamental principles, each contributing to its unique approach to healing:

a. **The Law of Similars**: This principle states that a substance capable of producing certain symptoms in a healthy person can be used to treat similar symptoms in a sick person. For example, if a substance causes fever and restlessness in a healthy individual, it can be used as a homeopathic remedy for someone experiencing those same symptoms due to illness.

b. **The Minimum Dose**: Homeopathic remedies are highly diluted, often to the point where there may be no molecules of the original substance left. This extreme dilution is believed to enhance the remedy's healing properties while minimizing any potential toxicity.

c. **Individualization**: Homeopathy recognizes that each person is unique, and the same illness can manifest differently in different individuals. Treatment is tailored to the specific symptoms, emotional state, and overall constitution of the patient. Homeopaths conduct detailed interviews to understand the patient's complete symptom picture.

d. **Vital Force and Healing**: Homeopathy acknowledges the presence of a vital force or life energy within the body. When this vital force is in balance, the body is healthy. Disease is seen as a disturbance in this vital force, and homeopathic remedies are thought to stimulate the body's innate healing ability, helping it regain equilibrium.

e. **Holistic Approach**: Homeopathy considers the totality of symptoms, including physical, mental, and emotional aspects, when selecting a remedy. The emotional state of the patient, their likes and dislikes, and other seemingly unrelated factors are taken into account to choose the most appropriate remedy.

f. **Miasmatic Theory**: Homeopathy also incorporates the concept of miasms, which are inherited predispositions to certain diseases or susceptibilities. Treating underlying miasms is considered essential for long-term healing.

In practice, a homeopath carefully selects a remedy that matches the patient's unique symptom profile. The remedy is then administered in the belief that it will stimulate the body's vital force to restore balance and trigger the innate healing process. The response to homeopathic treatment varies from person to person, with some experiencing rapid improvement and others requiring longer-term care.

It's important to note that while many people report positive experiences with homeopathy, its mechanisms of action remain a subject of debate and ongoing research. Critics argue that the extreme dilutions used in homeopathy render remedies biologically implausible, while proponents point to clinical outcomes as evidence of its efficacy.

Homeopathy is a holistic and individualized system of medicine rooted in the principle of "like cures like." Its history, dating back to Samuel Hahnemann's discoveries in the late 18th century, has seen it evolve and endure as a complementary or alternative approach to health and healing. Its unique principles, including potentization and individualization, guide the selection and administration of highly diluted remedies with the aim of stimulating the body's vital force and promoting overall well-being. While it remains a subject of debate and research, homeopathy continues to be embraced by individuals seeking gentle and holistic approaches to healthcare.

CHAPTER 2

Principles of Homeopathy

2.1 The Law of Similars

The Law of Similars, often referred to as "similia similibus curentur" in Latin, is the foundational principle of homeopathy. It states that a substance capable of producing specific symptoms in a healthy person can be used to treat similar symptoms in a sick person. In other words, "like cures like."

This principle was first observed by Samuel Hahnemann, the founder of homeopathy, during his experimentation with various substances on himself and others. He noticed that when he ingested certain substances that caused symptoms similar to those of certain diseases, the substances could alleviate the symptoms of those diseases. For instance, cinchona bark, which contains quinine and can induce symptoms similar to malaria, was found to be effective in treating malaria.

To apply the Law of Similars in practice, a homeopathic practitioner carefully evaluates a patient's symptoms, taking into account not only the physical complaints but also the patient's emotional state, preferences, and unique manifestations of the illness. The goal is to find a homeopathic remedy that matches the totality of the patient's symptoms as closely as possible.

2.2 The Minimum Dose

The Minimum Dose principle emphasizes the use of highly diluted remedies in homeopathy. Hahnemann recognized that many substances that could cure diseases in their crude, concentrated forms could also be toxic or produce undesirable side effects. To overcome this challenge, he developed a process known as potentization.

Potentization involves serial dilution and succussion (vigorous shaking) of a remedy to the point where the original substance becomes extremely diluted, often to the point where no molecules of the original substance may remain in the final remedy. Paradoxically, as the remedy is diluted further, its curative power is believed to increase while its toxicity diminishes.

The process of potentization is typically denoted by a number and a letter, such as 6C or 30X. The number represents the number of serial dilutions, and the letter (C or X) indicates the scale of dilution. For example, a 6C remedy has undergone six serial dilutions of 1:100, while a 30X remedy has undergone 30 serial dilutions of 1:10.

Homeopaths believe that this extreme dilution process activates the vital energy or "vital force" of the substance, making it a safe and effective treatment. This aligns with the concept that less is often more in homeopathy, and the healing effect is potentiated by the energetic imprint of the original substance.

2.3 Individualization

Individualization is a crucial aspect of homeopathic practice. Homeopaths recognize that each person is unique, and the same disease or health condition can manifest differently in different individuals. Therefore, homeopathic treatment is highly personalized and tailored to the individual patient.

To achieve individualization, homeopathic practitioners conduct thorough and detailed consultations with their patients. They gather information not only about the physical symptoms but also about the patient's mental and emotional state, lifestyle, and even their likes and dislikes. This comprehensive assessment helps create a complete "symptom picture" of the patient.

The goal is to select a homeopathic remedy that closely matches the totality of the patient's symptoms, both physical and emotional. This remedy is believed to stimulate the body's innate healing ability, addressing the root causes of the illness rather than just alleviating the symptoms.

Individualization is one of the key reasons why two individuals with the same medical diagnosis may receive different homeopathic remedies. Homeopaths consider the whole person when prescribing remedies, aiming to restore balance and harmony on a deep level, leading to long-term healing and well-being.

The principles of homeopathy encompass the Law of Similars, which dictates that like cures like; the Minimum Dose, emphasizing extreme dilution to enhance remedy safety and efficacy; and Individualization, which tailors' treatment to the unique symptom picture and constitution of each individual patient. These principles collectively form the core of homeopathic practice, guiding the selection and administration of remedies with the goal of stimulating the body's natural healing mechanisms.

2.4 Vital Force and Healing

Central to homeopathy's philosophy and principles is the concept of the "vital force" (also known as the "vital energy" or "life force"). This concept is integral to understanding how homeopathy perceives the process of healing.

In homeopathy, it is believed that every living organism possesses a vital force or energy that animates and sustains life. This vital force maintains the body's balance and equilibrium, ensuring proper functioning and health. When the vital force is in harmony, an individual experiences good health and well-being.

However, illnesses and diseases are seen as disruptions or imbalances in this vital force. Homeopathy postulates that symptoms of illness are the body's way of expressing this disturbance in the vital force. These symptoms manifest not as the disease itself but as the body's attempt to restore balance and eliminate the underlying disturbance.

The role of the homeopathic remedy is to stimulate and support the vital force in its efforts to restore equilibrium. Remedies are chosen based on the principle of "like cures like" (Law of Similars), as described earlier. The remedy, when closely matched to the patient's symptom picture, is believed to resonate with the vital force and initiate a healing response.

Homeopaths often describe this process as "energetic" or "dynamic" healing. The remedy is thought to work at a deep level, addressing the underlying energetic imbalance rather than merely suppressing or masking symptoms. It is believed to gently nudge the vital force back into harmony, allowing the body to heal itself.

The concept of vital force in homeopathy aligns with the idea that the body has a remarkable capacity for self-healing. Rather than relying solely on external interventions, homeopathy seeks to support and enhance the body's innate healing abilities. This approach aims to promote not only the resolution of current health issues but also an overall improvement in a person's vitality and well-being.

Critics of homeopathy often question the existence of the vital force and its role in healing, as these concepts are difficult to measure or quantify using conventional scientific methods. However, proponents of homeopathy maintain that the success of homeopathic treatment, as reported by many patients and practitioners, is evidence of its effectiveness in working with the vital force to achieve healing and balance.

The concept of the vital force is a fundamental element of homeopathy's approach to healing. It posits that illnesses and symptoms are reflections of disturbances in the body's vital force, and homeopathic remedies, chosen through the Law of Similars, are believed to resonate with and support the vital force in its efforts to restore health. While the concept may be debated from a scientific perspective, it remains a cornerstone of homeopathic philosophy and practice.

CHAPTER 3

Homeopathic Remedies

3.1 Homeopathic Remedies: Selection and Preparation

Homeopathic remedies are central to homeopathic treatment, and their selection and preparation are key aspects of homeopathic practice.

Selection of Remedies:

- Homeopathic remedies are derived from various sources, including plants, minerals, animals, and even certain chemical compounds.

- The selection of a remedy is based on the principle of "like cures like" (Law of Similars). Homeopaths match the patient's symptoms as closely as possible to the known symptom picture of a remedy.

- Homeopaths conduct detailed interviews and assessments to gather information about the patient's physical symptoms, mental and emotional state, and overall constitution.

- The goal is to find a remedy that encompasses the totality of the patient's symptoms, both the specific ailment and the broader picture of their health.

Preparation of Remedies:

- Homeopathic remedies are prepared through a unique

process called potentization, which involves a series of dilutions and succussions (vigorous shaking).

- The starting material, such as a plant extract or mineral, is first dissolved in alcohol or water to create a mother tincture.

- The mother tincture is then diluted repeatedly, often to an extreme degree. With each dilution, the remedy is succussed, believed to transfer the vital energy of the substance into the solution.

- Homeopathic remedies are typically labeled with a potency, indicating the number of serial dilutions and succussions. Common potencies include 6C, 30X, 200C, etc.

- The final remedy may be in the form of small sugar pellets (globules) or liquid drops.

3.2 Common Remedies

Homeopathy boasts a wide range of remedies, each derived from a different source and suited to specific symptom profiles. While there are hundreds of remedies, here are some examples of common homeopathic remedies and the conditions they are often used to treat:

- **Arnica montana**: Arnica is used for bruising, muscle soreness, and trauma. It is often used after accidents, surgery, or physical overexertion.

- **Belladonna**: Belladonna is employed for sudden, intense fevers, redness, and heat. It may be used for conditions with throbbing pain, such as headaches.

- **Apis mellifica**: Apis is used for bee-sting-like pains, swelling, and burning sensations. It's often chosen for conditions involving edema or allergic reactions.

- **Ignatia**: Ignatia is associated with emotional distress, grief, and hysteria. It may be used for individuals who experience mood swings or sudden emotional upsets.

- **Nux vomica**: Nux vomica is used for digestive issues, particularly those related to overindulgence, such as indigestion, heartburn, and constipation.

- **Pulsatilla**: Pulsatilla is often indicated for people with changeable moods, mild temperament, and symptoms that shift from one part of the body to another. It's used for conditions like colds, coughs, and menstrual problems.

- **Rhus toxicodendron**: Rhus tox is used for conditions involving stiffness and restlessness, such as rheumatism or poison ivy rashes.

homeopathic remedies are chosen based on the individual's unique symptom profile, and what works for one person may not be suitable for another, even if they have a similar condition.

3.3 Potencies and Dilutions

The potency and dilution of a homeopathic remedy are significant factors in its selection and effectiveness:

- **Low Potencies (e.g., 6C, 12C):** These potencies are considered mild and are often used for acute conditions with strong, well-defined symptoms. They are generally safe for self-administration.

- **Medium Potencies (e.g., 30C):** Medium potencies are versatile and are commonly used for a wide range of acute and chronic conditions. They are often selected when the exact remedy is known but the symptom picture is not entirely clear.

- **High Potencies (e.g., 200C, 1M, 10M)**: High potencies are typically used for chronic and deep-seated conditions. They are chosen when the symptom picture closely matches the remedy and when the vital force needs a more powerful stimulus.

- **Ultra-High Potencies (e.g., 50M, CM)**: These potencies are very dilute and are reserved for complex or long-standing chronic conditions. They should be prescribed by experienced homeopaths.

The principle of "less is more" applies to homeopathic potencies. Higher potencies are more diluted and are believed to act more deeply on the vital force. The choice of potency is determined by the individual patient's condition and responsiveness to treatment.

Homeopathic remedies are selected and prepared based on the principle of "like cures like" and are chosen to match the patient's unique symptom profile. Common remedies are derived from various sources and are used for specific conditions. Potencies and dilutions are carefully considered to tailor the remedy to the individual's needs and the nature of their condition, with the goal of stimulating the vital force and promoting healing.

CHAPTER 4

Homeopathic Treatment

4.1 Consultation with a Homeopath

A consultation with a qualified homeopath is the first step in receiving homeopathic treatment. Homeopathic consultations are thorough, holistic, and individualized, allowing the practitioner to gain a comprehensive understanding of the patient's health and to select the most appropriate remedy.

Here's what you can expect during a consultation with a homeopath:

1. Detailed Case Taking:

- The homeopath will begin by asking about your chief complaint, the main reason you seek treatment. They will encourage you to describe your symptoms in detail, including their location, sensation, intensity, and any accompanying factors.

- Beyond the physical symptoms, the homeopath will inquire about your emotional and mental state. They may ask about your mood, fears, anxieties, stressors, and any recent life events.

- Lifestyle factors, such as diet, sleep patterns, exercise, and environmental factors, may also be discussed. Your preferences and aversions in terms of food, temperature, and other environmental factors may be important.

- Your medical history, including past illnesses, surgeries, and any medications or treatments you are currently using, will be explored.

2. Complete Symptom Picture:

- The homeopath will aim to create a complete "symptom picture" by understanding not only your current symptoms but also any recurring patterns or symptoms you've experienced throughout your life.

- The goal is to identify the unique expression of your

illness, including any unusual or uncommon symptoms, to match it with a specific homeopathic remedy.

3. Individualization:

- Homeopathy is highly individualized. The homeopath will consider your physical, emotional, and mental state as a whole, rather than focusing solely on the disease label.

- You'll be encouraged to express your feelings, experiences, and concerns openly, as this information helps the homeopath select a remedy that resonates with your unique constitution.

4. Physical Examination (if necessary):

- In some cases, a homeopath may conduct a physical examination to assess specific symptoms or conditions. This could include examining your skin, nails, tongue, or other physical signs related to your health.

5. Selection of Homeopathic Remedy:

- Based on the information gathered during the consultation, the homeopath will carefully select a homeopathic remedy that closely matches your overall symptom picture.

- The remedy is chosen following the principle of "like cures like" (Law of Similars). It is believed that the remedy, when administered in a highly diluted form, will stimulate your vital force to initiate the healing process.

6. Dosage and Follow-Up:

- The homeopath will provide specific instructions on how to take the remedy, including dosage and timing.

- You will be advised on any lifestyle or dietary changes that may complement the treatment.

- Follow-up appointments will be scheduled to assess your progress and make any necessary adjustments to the treatment plan. Homeopathy often involves a series of follow-up consultations to track changes and refine the treatment as needed.

7. Holistic Approach:

- Homeopaths consider not only the specific symptoms but also the underlying causes and contributing factors to your condition. This holistic approach aims to address the root causes of illness and promote overall well-being.

8. Open Communication:

- Throughout the treatment process, open and honest communication with your homeopath is essential. You should report any changes in your symptoms, emotional state, or overall well-being, as this information guides the adjustment of the remedy.

seek out a qualified and registered homeopath who has undergone formal training and is recognized by a reputable homeopathic organization. During the consultation, you should feel comfortable sharing your health concerns and experiences, as this information is crucial for the homeopath to provide effective and individualized treatment. Homeopathy is generally considered safe and can be used alongside conventional medical care, but it's advisable to inform your healthcare providers of any homeopathic treatments you are receiving to ensure coordinated care.

4.2 Case Taking and Analysis

Case taking and analysis are critical steps in the homeopathic treatment process, ensuring that the selected remedy is the most appropriate match for the patient's unique symptom profile. Here's an overview of these essential aspects:

Case Taking:

- Case taking is the process of collecting detailed information about the patient's physical, mental, and emotional symptoms, as well as their overall constitution and life circumstances.

- The homeopath conducts a comprehensive interview, asking questions about the patient's chief complaint, symptoms, and the factors that exacerbate or alleviate their condition.

- The patient's emotional state, temperament, personality traits, and responses to stress are explored.

- Lifestyle factors, such as diet, sleep patterns, exercise, and environmental influences, are considered.

- Past medical history, family medical history, and any medications or treatments the patient is currently using are reviewed.

- Specifics about any recent or ongoing life events, traumas, or emotional stressors may be discussed.

Analysis:

- Once the case-taking process is complete, the homeopath carefully analyzes the information gathered to form a complete and detailed symptom picture.

- The goal is to identify the characteristic and unique symptoms that differentiate the patient's experience from others with similar conditions.

- Common symptoms, as well as unusual or peculiar symptoms, are taken into account, as homeopathy places great importance on individualizing treatment based on these characteristics.

- The homeopath considers the totality of the symptoms, including the physical, mental, and emotional aspects, to find a remedy that closely matches this unique symptom picture.

Repertorization:

- Homeopaths often use
  reportories, which are
  specialized reference books or
  software programs, to help
  identify potential remedies.

- A repertory contains a vast list
  of symptoms and their
  associated remedies. The
  homeopath selects symptoms
  from the patient's case and
  looks for remedies that match
  those symptoms in the
  repertory.

- The repertorization process
  helps narrow down the list of
  possible remedies that closely
  correspond to the patient's
  symptoms.

Materia Medica:

- The homeopath refers to
  materia medica, which is a

comprehensive compilation of information about individual homeopathic remedies.

- Materia medica provides detailed descriptions of each remedy's symptom picture, including the physical, mental, and emotional characteristics it is known to address.

- By comparing the patient's symptom picture with the descriptions in the materia medica, the homeopath can further refine the remedy selection.

4.3 Treatment Plans

Once the homeopath has gathered, analyzed, and repertorized the patient's case, they will formulate a treatment plan tailored to the individual's needs. Here are the key components of a homeopathic treatment plan:

Remedy Selection:

- The homeopath selects a homeopathic remedy that best matches the patient's unique symptom picture, considering the Law of Similars.

- The potency (dilution) and dosage of the remedy are determined based on the individual's sensitivity and the nature of their condition.

Dosage and Administration:

- The homeopath provides clear instructions on how to take the remedy, including the number of pellets or drops, frequency of dosing, and any specific guidelines (e.g., avoiding certain substances like coffee or mint).

- Patients are often advised to take the remedy away from meals to ensure optimal absorption.

Follow-Up Appointments:

- Homeopathic treatment typically involves a series of follow-up appointments to monitor progress and make any necessary adjustments to the treatment plan.

- The frequency of follow-up appointments varies depending on the patient's condition and the homeopath's assessment.

Lifestyle and Dietary Guidance:

- Homeopaths may provide recommendations for dietary and lifestyle modifications that support the healing process.

- Patients may be advised to make changes in their habits or environment to promote overall well-being.

Monitoring and Assessment:

- During follow-up appointments, the homeopath evaluates the patient's response to the remedy, including changes in symptoms, emotional state, and overall health.

- Adjustments to the remedy or treatment plan may be made based on the patient's progress.

Long-Term Care:

- For chronic or complex conditions, homeopathic treatment may extend over an extended period.

- The goal is to not only alleviate immediate symptoms but also address underlying imbalances and promote long-term health.

homeopathy is highly individualized, and treatment plans are tailored to each patient's specific needs. The homeopath's expertise lies in selecting remedies that resonate with the patient's unique symptom picture, ultimately supporting the body's self-healing mechanisms and restoring balance. Open communication and collaboration between the patient and the homeopath are key to the success of homeopathic treatment.

4.4 Managing Acute and Chronic Conditions

Homeopathy can be used to manage a wide range of health conditions, both acute and chronic. The approach to treatment may differ depending on the nature and duration of the condition. Here's an overview of how homeopathy is used to manage acute and chronic conditions:

Managing Acute Conditions:

1. **Rapid Symptom Relief:** Homeopathy is well-suited for acute conditions that have sudden and intense symptoms, such as fevers, colds, flu, injuries, and acute digestive issues. The goal is to provide rapid relief by selecting a remedy that closely matches the

patient's acute symptom picture.

2. **Individualized Treatment:** Even in acute cases, homeopaths consider the individual's unique symptom presentation. They take into account the specific nature of the symptoms, such as the type of pain, location, sensation, and modalities (factors that worsen or alleviate symptoms). This individualization helps in selecting the most appropriate remedy.

3. **Prompt Administration:** Remedies for acute conditions are typically administered frequently, often every 15 minutes to an hour, until there is improvement. As symptoms improve, the frequency of

remedy administration may decrease.

4. **Monitoring Progress:** Patients are advised to closely monitor their symptoms and report any changes to the homeopath. Adjustments to the remedy or dosing may be made based on the patient's response.

5. **Self-Care:** In many cases, homeopaths empower patients to use acute remedies at home for common, self-limiting conditions. Patients may be provided with a homeopathic first-aid kit and instructions on how to use remedies for minor injuries and ailments.

6. **Integration with Conventional Care:** Homeopathy can be used

alongside conventional medical care for acute conditions. It is essential to communicate with healthcare providers to ensure coordinated and safe treatment.

Managing Chronic Conditions:

1. **In-Depth Case Taking:** Chronic conditions often require a more thorough and comprehensive assessment of the patient's physical, mental, and emotional health. The homeopath delves into the patient's complete symptom picture, life history, and constitution.

2. **Treatment Plan Development:** Homeopaths develop a long-term treatment plan aimed at addressing the underlying causes of the

chronic condition. The goal is not only to alleviate symptoms but also to promote overall health and well-being.

3. **Individualized Treatment:** Homeopathic remedies for chronic conditions are selected based on the Law of Similars, matching the patient's unique symptom picture. The remedy's potency and dosing schedule are carefully chosen to stimulate the vital force gently.

4. **Regular Follow-Up:** Patients with chronic conditions typically have regular follow-up appointments with the homeopath to assess progress, adjust remedies, and refine the treatment plan.

5. **Lifestyle and Dietary Guidance:** Homeopaths may provide recommendations for lifestyle and dietary changes that support the healing process. These changes are often individualized to the patient's specific needs.

6. **Integrated Approach:** Homeopathy can be used as a standalone treatment for chronic conditions or as a complementary therapy alongside conventional medicine. It is crucial for patients to inform their healthcare providers about their homeopathic treatment to ensure safe and coordinated care.

7. **Long-Term Management:** Chronic conditions may require

long-term homeopathic treatment. The goal is to improve the patient's quality of life, reduce the frequency and severity of symptoms, and support the body's innate healing abilities.

8. **Monitoring Progress:** The patient and homeopath work collaboratively to monitor the progress of the treatment. Adjustments to the remedy and treatment plan are made based on the patient's response and changing symptom patterns.

recognize that homeopathy takes a holistic and individualized approach to both acute and chronic conditions. The choice of remedies, dosages, and treatment duration is tailored to the unique needs of each patient. While homeopathy may not be a replacement for all aspects of conventional medical care, it can be a valuable complement in managing a wide range of health conditions.

CHAPTER 5

Conditions Treated with Homeopathy

5.1 Respiratory Issues

Homeopathy is frequently used to treat a variety of respiratory issues, both acute and chronic. It can provide relief from symptoms and support the body's natural healing processes. Here are some common respiratory conditions that may be treated with homeopathy:

1. **Common Colds and Flu**: Homeopathic remedies can help alleviate symptoms like congestion, runny nose, cough, and fever associated with colds and flu.

2. **Asthma**: Homeopathy may be used to manage asthma symptoms, including wheezing, shortness of breath, and coughing. Individualized treatment aims to reduce the frequency and severity of asthma attacks.

3. **Bronchitis**: Homeopathic remedies can help soothe coughing, reduce chest discomfort, and promote recovery in acute bronchitis. For chronic bronchitis, constitutional treatment may be necessary.

4. **Allergic Rhinitis (Hay Fever)**: Homeopathy offers relief from hay fever symptoms like sneezing, itchy eyes, and nasal congestion. Remedies are selected based on the specific

allergens triggering the symptoms.

5. **Sinusitis**: Homeopathy can address symptoms of sinusitis, such as facial pain, congestion, and headaches. Constitutional treatment may be recommended for recurrent or chronic sinusitis.

6. **Tonsillitis and Sore Throat**: Remedies may help reduce pain and inflammation associated with tonsillitis and sore throats. Specific remedies are chosen based on the nature of the throat discomfort.

7. **Respiratory Infections**: Homeopathy can be used to support the body's immune response and speed up recovery from respiratory infections,

such as pneumonia and bronchopneumonia.

8. **Chronic Obstructive Pulmonary Disease (COPD)**: Homeopathic treatment may be integrated with conventional care to improve the quality of life for COPD patients by reducing breathlessness and enhancing overall well-being.

5.2 Digestive Disorders

Homeopathy can be effective in addressing a wide range of digestive disorders, from acute conditions like indigestion to chronic conditions such as irritable bowel syndrome (IBS). Here are some digestive disorders that may benefit from homeopathic treatment:

1. **Indigestion**: Homeopathic remedies can provide relief from symptoms of indigestion, such as bloating, acidity, and discomfort after eating.

2. **Acid Reflux (GERD)**: Homeopathy offers remedies to reduce heartburn, regurgitation, and other symptoms associated with gastroesophageal reflux disease (GERD).

3. **Irritable Bowel Syndrome (IBS)**: Homeopathy can help manage the symptoms of IBS, including abdominal pain, diarrhea, constipation, and bloating. Constitutional treatment is often used for long-term relief.

4. **Diarrhea**: Homeopathic remedies can be used to address

acute and chronic diarrhea,
balancing the digestive system
and restoring normal bowel
movements.

5. **Constipation**: Homeopathy
   provides remedies to relieve
   constipation by promoting
   regular bowel movements and
   alleviating discomfort.

6. **Gallbladder Disorders**:
   Conditions like gallstones or
   inflammation of the gallbladder
   (cholecystitis) may be managed
   with homeopathy to reduce
   pain and inflammation.

7. **Peptic Ulcers**: Homeopathy
   can help soothe symptoms of
   peptic ulcers, such as
   abdominal pain, burning
   sensation, and nausea.

8. **Food Allergies and Sensitivities**: Homeopathy can be used to address symptoms related to food allergies and sensitivities, such as skin rashes, digestive upset, and respiratory symptoms.

9. **Inflammatory Bowel Disease (IBD)**: While homeopathy may not cure IBD, it may help manage symptoms and improve the patient's overall well-being in conjunction with conventional medical care.

homeopathic treatment for digestive disorders is highly individualized, with remedies chosen based on the patient's specific symptoms and constitution. Homeopathy aims to address the root causes of digestive issues and promote balance in the digestive system, leading to improved overall health and well-being. As with any medical condition, individuals should consult with a qualified homeopath or healthcare provider for an accurate diagnosis and tailored treatment plan.

5.3 Skin Conditions

Homeopathy is often utilized to treat various skin conditions, offering both relief from symptoms and support for long-term healing. Here are some common skin conditions that may benefit from homeopathic treatment:

1. **Eczema (Dermatitis)**: Homeopathic remedies can help alleviate itching, inflammation, and redness associated with eczema. Individualized treatment aims to address the underlying causes of flare-ups.

2. **Psoriasis**: Homeopathy may provide relief from the symptoms of psoriasis, including scaling, itching, and skin thickening. Constitutional treatment is often employed for chronic cases.

3. **Acne**: Homeopathic remedies can target the underlying factors contributing to acne, such as hormonal imbalances or digestive issues. Treatment is tailored to the patient's specific acne type and triggers.

4. **Urticaria (Hives)**: Homeopathy offers remedies to reduce the itching and swelling of hives. Specific remedies are chosen based on the trigger of the allergic reaction.

5. **Vitiligo**: While vitiligo is a complex condition, homeopathic treatment may help slow its progression and improve pigmentation in some cases.

6. **Boils and Abscesses**: Homeopathic remedies can promote the healing of boils and abscesses by reducing pain, inflammation, and the tendency to recur.

7. **Fungal Infections**: Conditions like ringworm and athlete's foot may respond to homeopathic antifungal remedies, which can be used alongside conventional treatments.

8. **Herpes (Cold Sores and Genital Herpes)**: Homeopathy may help reduce the frequency

and severity of herpes outbreaks and alleviate associated symptoms.

9. **Warts**: Homeopathic remedies can be applied topically to warts or used internally to stimulate the body's immune response to the virus causing warts.

5.4 Musculoskeletal Problems

Homeopathy can be effective in managing a range of musculoskeletal issues, providing relief from pain and promoting healing. Here are some conditions in this category:

1. **Arthritis**: Homeopathic remedies are used to manage pain, stiffness, and

inflammation associated with various types of arthritis, including osteoarthritis and rheumatoid arthritis.

2. **Muscle Sprains and Strains**: Homeopathy may help reduce pain and swelling in acute injuries and support the healing of damaged muscle fibers.

3. **Back Pain**: Homeopathic remedies can target different types of back pain, such as sciatica, herniated discs, or muscle spasms, providing relief and promoting recovery.

4. **Gout**: Homeopathy may help manage the symptoms of gout, such as severe joint pain and inflammation.

5. **Fibromyalgia**: While fibromyalgia is a complex

condition, homeopathy may offer relief from some of the associated symptoms, including widespread pain, fatigue, and sleep disturbances.

6. **Tendonitis**: Homeopathy can be used to reduce inflammation and pain in tendons affected by conditions like Achilles tendonitis or tennis elbow.

7. **Frozen Shoulder (Adhesive Capsulitis)**: Homeopathic remedies may help relieve pain and improve the range of motion in cases of frozen shoulder.

5.5 Emotional and Mental Health

Homeopathy is well-suited for addressing emotional and mental health concerns. It recognizes the connection between the mind and body and aims to restore balance on all levels. Here are some emotional and mental health issues that may be treated with homeopathy:

1. **Anxiety Disorders**: Homeopathic remedies can be used to alleviate symptoms of anxiety, such as restlessness, palpitations, and excessive worry. Individualized treatment considers the specific type of anxiety (e.g., social anxiety, generalized anxiety disorder).

2. **Depression**: Homeopathy may offer support for individuals

experiencing depression, addressing emotional symptoms like sadness, hopelessness, and changes in appetite or sleep patterns.

3. **Stress and Burnout**: Homeopathy can help manage stress-related symptoms, such as fatigue, irritability, and physical tension.

4. **Panic Attacks**: Homeopathic remedies may be used to reduce the frequency and intensity of panic attacks and alleviate associated symptoms like rapid heartbeat and shortness of breath.

5. **Obsessive-Compulsive Disorder (OCD)**: While OCD often requires a multidisciplinary approach,

homeopathy may help reduce the intensity of obsessive thoughts and compulsions.

6. **Attention-Deficit/Hyperactivity Disorder (ADHD)**: Homeopathy may be integrated with other treatments to address symptoms like hyperactivity, impulsivity, and inattention.

7. **Sleep Disorders**: Homeopathic remedies can support individuals with sleep disturbances, helping to improve the quality and duration of sleep.

8. **Phobias and Trauma**: Homeopathy may be used to address specific fears and phobias or to support individuals who have

experienced trauma by alleviating emotional and physical symptoms.

Homeopathic treatment for emotional and mental health conditions is highly individualized, with remedies chosen based on the patient's unique symptom profile and emotional state. It is often used as a complementary approach alongside other therapeutic modalities, including counseling or psychotherapy, to provide comprehensive care for emotional well-being. Patients should consult with a qualified homeopath or mental health professional for personalized treatment plans.

CHAPTER 6

Homeopathy for Daily Health

6.1 First Aid and Minor Injuries

Homeopathy is widely used for first aid and minor injuries, providing gentle and effective remedies for common household accidents and injuries. Here are some scenarios where homeopathy can be applied for first aid:

1. **Bruises and Contusions**: Homeopathic remedies like Arnica montana are frequently

used to reduce swelling and bruising after injuries. Arnica can also help relieve soreness and muscle pain.

2. **Sprains and Strains**: Remedies such as Rhus toxicodendron and Ruta graveolens can be used to alleviate pain, stiffness, and inflammation associated with sprained joints or strained muscles.

3. **Minor Burns**: Homeopathic remedies like Cantharis and Urtica urens can provide relief from pain and promote healing in cases of minor burns or scalds.

4. **Cuts and Abrasions**: Calendula is a well-known homeopathic remedy for cuts

and abrasions. It can help
cleanse wounds and stimulate
the healing process.

5. **Insect Bites and Stings**:
Remedies like Apis mellifica
and Ledum palustre are used to
reduce swelling, itching, and
discomfort caused by insect
bites and stings.

6. **Splinters**: Homeopathic
remedies like Silicea can help
expel splinters or foreign
objects embedded in the skin.

7. **Shock and Trauma**: Aconitum
napellus may be used in cases
of emotional shock or trauma,
providing comfort and stability
during the initial stages of
shock.

8. **Nosebleeds**: Remedies like
Phosphorus or Ferrum

phosphoricum can be used to stop nosebleeds.

9. **Toothaches**: Homeopathic remedies like Coffea cruda or Chamomilla can provide temporary relief from toothaches until dental care can be sought.

10. **Motion Sickness**: Remedies like Cocculus indicus or Nux vomica can be used to alleviate symptoms of motion sickness, such as nausea and dizziness.

For first aid purposes, homeopathic remedies are typically administered in low potencies, such as 6C or 30C. These remedies are safe for self-administration, but it's important to consult a healthcare professional if there are concerns about the severity of the injury or if symptoms persist.

6.2 Preventive Homeopathy

Preventive homeopathy, also known as constitutional or constitutional treatment, focuses on enhancing overall health and preventing illness. It is a proactive approach to maintaining well-being and addressing underlying imbalances in the body. Here's how preventive homeopathy works:

1. **Individualized Assessment**: A homeopath conducts a comprehensive assessment of the patient's physical, mental, and emotional health. This includes gathering information about the patient's medical history, family history, lifestyle, and overall constitution.

2. **Remedy Selection**: Based on the patient's unique symptom picture and constitution, the homeopath selects a constitutional remedy that best matches the individual's overall state of health and susceptibilities.

3. **Treatment Plan**: Preventive homeopathic treatment involves taking the constitutional remedy over an extended period. The goal is to support the body's natural balance and vitality, making it less susceptible to illness.

4. **Regular Follow-Up**: Patients who undergo preventive homeopathy have regular follow-up appointments with the homeopath to assess progress and make any

necessary adjustments to the treatment plan.

5. **Lifestyle and Dietary Guidance**: Homeopaths may offer recommendations for lifestyle modifications and dietary changes that align with the patient's constitution and health goals.

6. **Stress Management**: Preventive homeopathy may include strategies for managing stress and emotional well-being, as stress can impact overall health.

7. **Prevention of Chronic Conditions**: Preventive homeopathy aims to prevent the development of chronic health issues and promote a higher level of well-being.

preventive homeopathy is tailored to the individual and is not a one-size-fits-all approach. The constitutional remedy is chosen to address the patient's unique susceptibilities and overall health. While preventive homeopathy is often used for long-term well-being, it can also be applied to address specific health concerns by targeting the underlying causes of those concerns. Patients interested in preventive homeopathy should seek out a qualified and experienced homeopath for a personalized assessment and treatment plan.

6.3 Building Immunity with Homeopathy

Homeopathy can be a valuable tool for building and strengthening the immune system. It is based on the principle of enhancing the body's innate ability to defend against pathogens and maintain overall health. Here's how homeopathy can contribute to immune system support:

1. **Constitutional Treatment**: Homeopaths often begin by assessing an individual's overall constitution and susceptibility to illness. By identifying and addressing underlying imbalances in the body, homeopathic remedies can help improve the overall vitality and resilience of the immune system.

2. **Immune-Supportive Remedies**: Homeopathy offers a range of remedies that can be used to support the immune system. These remedies are chosen based on the

individual's specific symptoms and susceptibility to infections. Examples include Echinacea, Thuja occidentalis, and Silicea.

3. **Preventive Treatment**: Homeopathic remedies like Oscillococcinum are often used preventively during flu seasons or when exposed to sick individuals. These remedies aim to stimulate the immune system's response to potential pathogens.

4. **Treatment of Recurrent Infections**: Homeopathy can address recurring infections, such as frequent colds or urinary tract infections, by strengthening the immune response and addressing underlying predispositions.

5. **Allergic Conditions**:
   Homeopathic treatment can
   help manage allergic conditions
   like hay fever or asthma,
   reducing the body's reactivity to
   allergens and supporting the
   immune system's balance.

6. **Stress Reduction**: Chronic
   stress can weaken the immune
   system. Homeopathy may
   include remedies to address the
   physical and emotional effects
   of stress, helping the body
   better cope with daily
   pressures.

7. **Diet and Lifestyle Guidance**:
   Homeopaths may provide
   recommendations for dietary
   and lifestyle changes that
   support immune health. This
   includes proper nutrition,

regular exercise, and adequate sleep.

8. **Detoxification**: Homeopathic remedies can be used in detoxification protocols to help the body eliminate toxins and promote optimal immune function.

9. **Balancing Chronic Conditions**: For individuals with chronic health conditions, homeopathy aims to address the underlying issues, improve overall health, and boost the immune system's capacity to fight infections.

10. **Individualized Approach**: Homeopathy takes into account the unique symptom picture of each person. Remedies are selected based on the

individual's specific physical, mental, and emotional symptoms, ensuring a tailored approach to immune support.

work with a qualified and experienced homeopath for immune system support. Homeopathic treatment is highly individualized, and the choice of remedies and treatment plans varies from person to person. While homeopathy can be a valuable complement to overall health and well-being, it should not replace conventional medical interventions when necessary, such as vaccinations or antibiotics for serious infections. Homeopathy and conventional medicine can often work together to provide comprehensive healthcare.

CHAPTER 7

Integrating Homeopathy with Conventional Medicine

7.1 Communicating with Healthcare Providers

Integrating homeopathy with conventional medicine can be a safe and effective approach to healthcare. However, open communication with your healthcare providers is crucial to ensure that all aspects of your treatment are coordinated effectively. Here's how to communicate effectively with your healthcare team:

1. **Inform Your Primary Care Physician**: Let your primary care physician or specialist know that you are using homeopathy as part of your healthcare regimen. Provide them with details about the remedies you are taking and the conditions you are addressing with homeopathy.

2. **Share Your Health Goals**: Clearly communicate your health goals and expectations with your healthcare providers. Discuss why you have chosen to incorporate homeopathy into your care plan and what you hope to achieve.

3. **Ask Questions**: If you have concerns or questions about integrating homeopathy with conventional medicine, don't

hesitate to ask your healthcare providers for guidance. They can offer insights into potential benefits and limitations.

4. **Request Coordinated Care**: Whenever possible, request coordinated care between your homeopath and other healthcare providers. This ensures that all treatments are aligned with your overall health objectives.

5. **Provide Health Records**: Share your medical history, including any diagnoses, treatments, and medications, with both your homeopath and conventional healthcare providers. This information helps them make informed decisions about your care.

6. **Regular Check-Ins**: Schedule regular check-ins with your healthcare providers to monitor your progress. These appointments allow for adjustments to your treatment plan, whether homeopathic or conventional.

7.2 Combining Treatments Safely

Integrating homeopathy with conventional medicine can be done safely with attention to the following considerations:

1. **Qualified Practitioners**: Ensure that you are working with qualified and experienced practitioners in both homeopathy and conventional

medicine. They can provide guidance on the safe integration of treatments.

2. **Understand Treatment Goals**: Be clear about the goals of each treatment. Homeopathy often aims to address underlying causes and promote overall well-being, while conventional medicine may focus on symptom relief or disease management.

3. **Dosage and Timing**: Follow dosage instructions for homeopathic remedies carefully. It's important not to exceed recommended doses. Be mindful of timing—some remedies should be taken away from meals or other substances.

4. **Monitoring Progress**:
    Regularly monitor your
    progress with both
    homeopathic and conventional
    treatments. Report any changes
    in symptoms, side effects, or
    overall well-being to your
    healthcare providers.

5. **Be Patient**: Homeopathy often
    takes time to show its effects,
    especially in chronic
    conditions. Be patient and
    committed to the treatment
    plan.

6. **Safety First**: If you experience
    a sudden and severe health
    issue or an emergency,
    prioritize seeking immediate
    medical attention through
    conventional channels.
    Homeopathy may be
    complementary but is not a

replacement for urgent medical care.

7.3 Managing Medication Interactions

When integrating homeopathy with conventional medications, consider the following strategies to manage potential interactions:

1. **Consult a pharmacist**: Talk to a pharmacist about potential interactions between homeopathic remedies and prescription or over-the-counter medications. Pharmacists can provide valuable insights into drug interactions.

2. **Timing**: Take homeopathic remedies at a different time from conventional medications

whenever possible. This reduces the likelihood of direct interactions.

3. **Discuss with Your Healthcare Providers**: Share information about all the substances you are using, including homeopathic remedies and supplements, with your healthcare providers. They can assess potential interactions and adjust treatment plans if necessary.

4. **Individualized Assessment**: The risk of interactions can vary depending on the specific medications and remedies involved, as well as individual factors. Discuss your unique situation with your healthcare team.

5. **Monitor for Side Effects**: Be vigilant for any unexpected side effects or changes in your health when combining treatments. Report any concerns to your healthcare providers promptly.

6. **Keep Records**: Maintain a detailed record of the remedies and medications you are using, including dosages and frequencies. This record can help healthcare providers assess your treatment plan effectively.

7. **Adhere to Instructions**: Follow dosing instructions for all treatments meticulously. This reduces the likelihood of overmedication or improper administration.

while there may be potential interactions between homeopathic remedies and conventional medications, the actual risk depends on individual circumstances. By working closely with your healthcare providers and being proactive in managing your healthcare, you can safely integrate homeopathy with conventional medicine to support your overall well-being.

CHAPTER 8

Safety and Side Effects

8.1 Homeopathy and Allergies

Homeopathic remedies are highly diluted and generally considered safe. However, individuals with allergies to specific substances used in homeopathic preparations should exercise caution. Here's what you need to know about homeopathy and allergies:

1. **Common Allergens**: Some homeopathic remedies are prepared from substances that could trigger allergies in

sensitive individuals. Common allergenic substances include plants (such as ragweed or poison ivy), animal products, and minerals.

2. **Consult a Homeopath**: If you have known allergies or are concerned about potential allergens in homeopathic remedies, consult a qualified homeopath. They can help you select remedies that are less likely to trigger allergic reactions.

3. **Homeopathic Consultation**: During a homeopathic consultation, inform your homeopath about any allergies or sensitivities you have. They will consider this information when recommending remedies.

4. **Safety Measures**: When trying
   a new homeopathic remedy,
   start with a low potency
   (dilution) to minimize the risk
   of allergic reactions. Observe
   your body's response and
   discontinue use if you
   experience any adverse effects.

5. **Allergen Labeling**: In some
   countries, regulations require
   homeopathic products to label
   potential allergens. Check
   product labels for any warnings
   related to allergens.

6. **Self-Administration**: If you
   are using over-the-counter
   homeopathic remedies and have
   known allergies, read product
   labels carefully and avoid those
   that contain allergens to which
   you are sensitive.

7. **Consult an Allergist**: If you
    suspect you may be allergic to a
    specific homeopathic remedy or
    substance, consult an allergist
    for testing and guidance.

8.2 Controversies and Criticisms

Homeopathy has been the subject of controversies and criticisms, primarily due to the following reasons:

1. **Scientific Skepticism**: Critics
    argue that homeopathy lacks
    scientific evidence to support
    its principles and efficacy. They
    contend that highly diluted
    remedies may not contain any
    active ingredients.

2. **Placebo Effect**: Some believe
    that the perceived benefits of

homeopathic treatments are mainly due to the placebo effect—the belief that the treatment will work rather than its actual properties.

3. **Safety Concerns**: Critics express concerns about the safety of homeopathic remedies, particularly when they are used as alternatives to conventional medicine in serious or life-threatening conditions.

4. **Regulation and Labeling**: There have been concerns about the regulation and labeling of homeopathic products, with critics suggesting that there may be inconsistencies in product quality and safety.

5. **Ethical Issues**: The use of homeopathy as a sole treatment for serious conditions can raise ethical concerns, as it may delay or prevent individuals from seeking evidence-based medical care.

approach homeopathy with a critical but open mind, considering the individual needs and preferences of each person. While some individuals report positive experiences with homeopathy, others may not find it effective for their health concerns. As with any healthcare approach, it's advisable to consult with qualified healthcare providers and make informed decisions based on your unique circumstances.

8.3 Ensuring Safe Practices

To ensure safe practices when using homeopathy, follow these guidelines:

1. **Consult a Qualified Homeopath**: Seek guidance from a qualified and experienced homeopath for a personalized assessment and treatment plan.

2. **Inform Your Healthcare Providers**: Inform your primary care physician and specialists about your use of homeopathic remedies, especially if you have underlying medical conditions or are taking prescription medications.

3. **Respect Conventional Medicine**: While homeopathy can be complementary, it should not replace conventional medical care, especially for serious or life-threatening conditions.

4. **Be Cautious with Allergies**: If you have known allergies, consult a homeopath and read product labels carefully to avoid potential allergens in homeopathic remedies.

5. **Start with Low Potency**: When trying a new remedy, start with a low potency to minimize the risk of adverse effects.

6. **Observe Changes and Side Effects**: Pay attention to any changes in your health or

unexpected side effects while using homeopathic remedies. Report any concerns to your healthcare providers.

7. **Select Reputable Products**: If using over-the-counter homeopathic products, choose reputable brands with good manufacturing practices and clear labeling.

8. **Critical Thinking**: Approach homeopathy with critical thinking, seeking information and evidence to make informed decisions about its use.